I0412229

My Alphabet Book of Fruits & Veggies

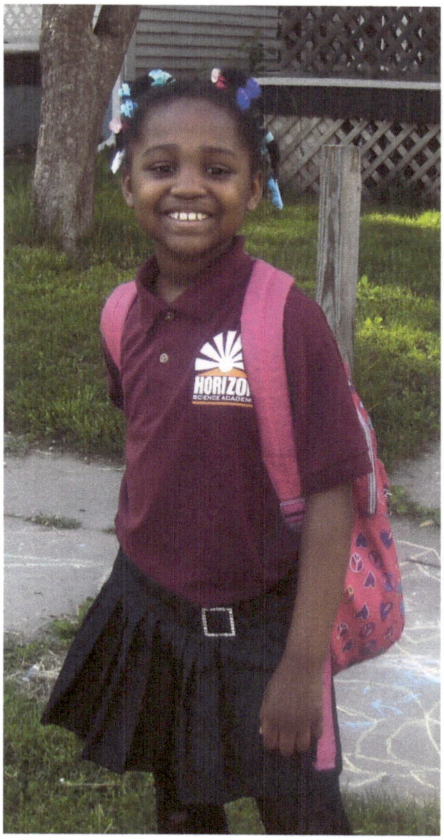

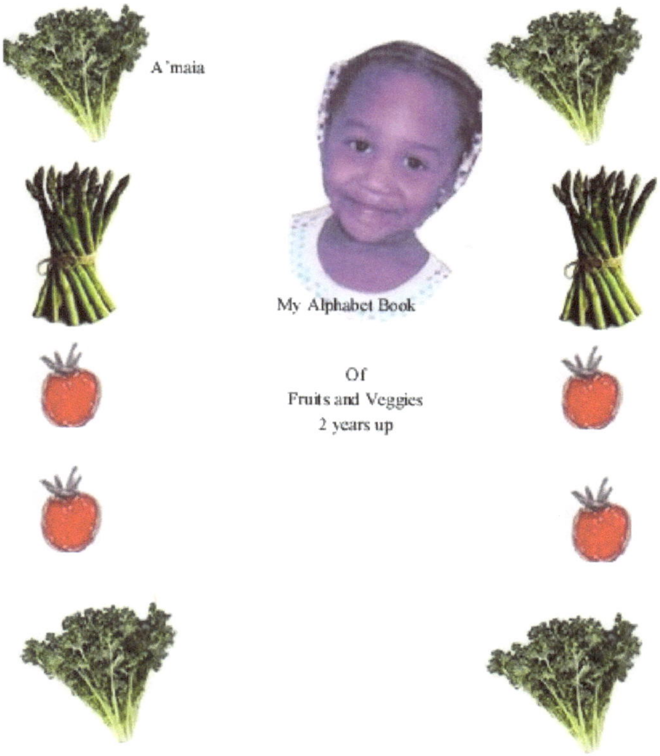

A 'maia

My Alphabet Book

Of
Fruits and Veggies
2 years up

By Mae Gardner-Blair
With a little help from the daycare kids

My Alphabet of Fruits & Veggies © 2013, Mae Blair. All rights reserved. No part of this book may be reproduced in any form or by any electronic or mechanical means without permission in writing from the publisher, except by a reviewer, who may quote brief passages in a review.

WORD LIST

ENGLISH	SPANISH
Asparagus	Esparrago
Broccoli	Brecol
Carrot	Zanahoria
Dandelion	Diente de leon
Egg Plant	Berenjena

Look at me eating broccoli

ENGLISH	SPANISH
Fennel	Hinojo
Garlic	Ajo
Habanero Pepper	Havana Pepper
Indian Corn	Indico Maiz
Jack Bean	frijoles del goto
Kale	Rizada
Lettuce	Lechuga

Is ice cream a vegetable?

ENGLISH	SPANISH
Mushroom	Seta

ENGLISH	SPANISH
Nectarine	Nectarina
Onion	Cebolla
Potato	Patata
Quince	Membrillo
Radish	Rabano
Squash	Calabaza
Tomato	Tomate
Ugli	Fruta de ugli
Voavanga	No translation
Watermelon	Sandia
Xigua	No translation
Yams	batata
Zucchini	Calabacin

Do I have to eat this, Granny?

Aa

Asparagus

English   Spanish

One = 1 ....Uno = 1

One serving of asparagus has only 20 calories, no fat or cholesterol, 5 mg. of sodium, 400 mg. of potassium, 5 grams of fiber, 60% of the USRDA of folacin, which is necessary for the formation of blood cells, growth, and prevention of liver disease.

Asparagus was first cultivated about 2500 years ago in Greece. In their conquests, the Romans spread it to the Gauls, Germans, Britons, and from there the rest of the world.

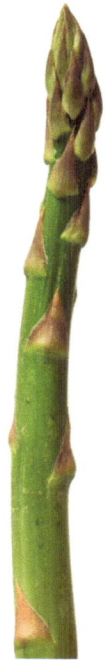

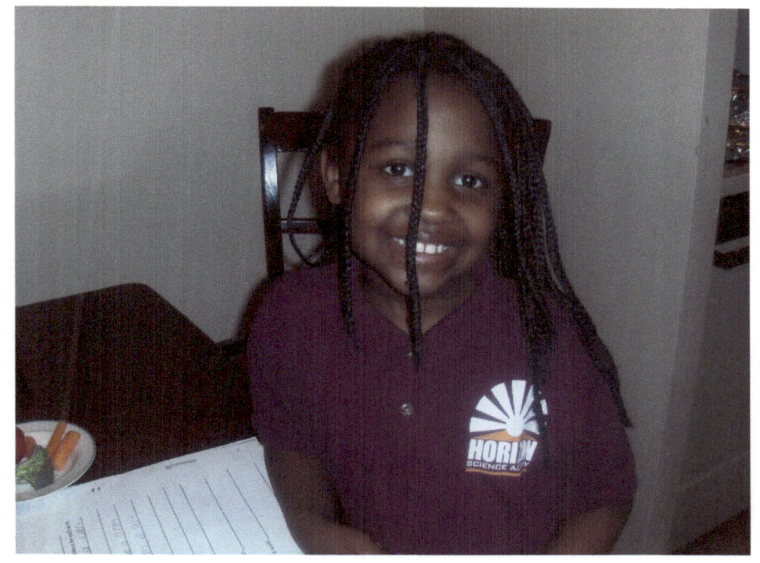

Who, me? Eat asparagus?

Bb

Broccoli

English	Spanish
Two = 2	Dos = 2

Broccoli gives us nutrition and helps our body fight diseases. This vegetable is high in vitamin C and dietary fiber. A single serving of broccoli provides 30 mg of vitamin C.

Broccoli also contains multiple nutrients with potent anti-cancer properties.

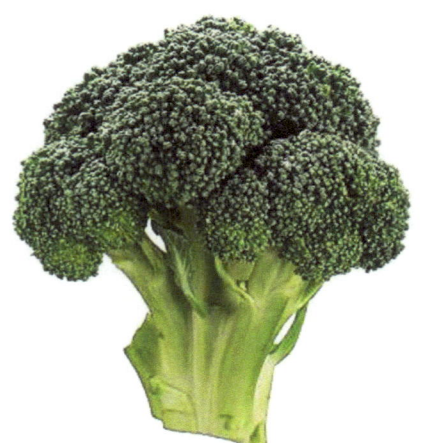

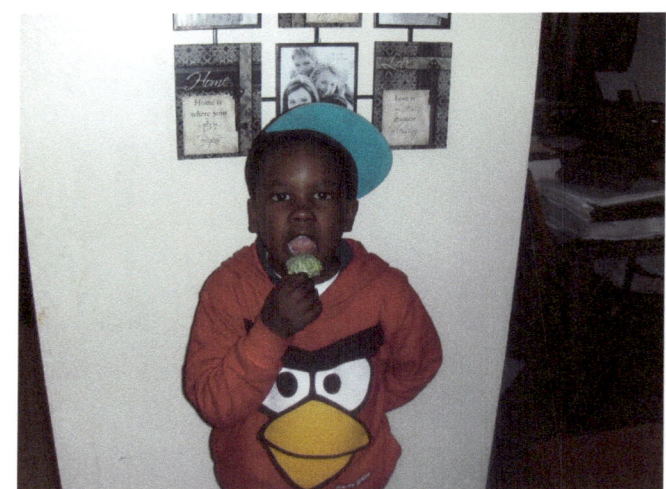

Okay, I'm eating it, Granny

Cc

Carrot

English	Spanish
Three = 3	Tres = 3

Carrots provide us with nutrients for healthy hair, eyes, skin, bones and mucous membranes.

The carrot gets its bright orange color from beta-carotene. Alpha and beta carotenes are partly metabolized into vitamin A in humans. Good for Bugs Bunny, good for kids.

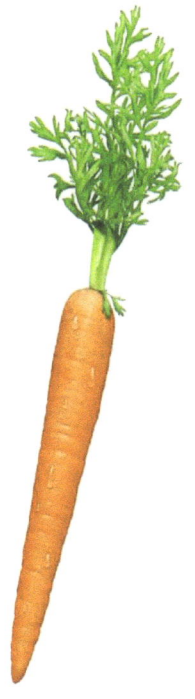

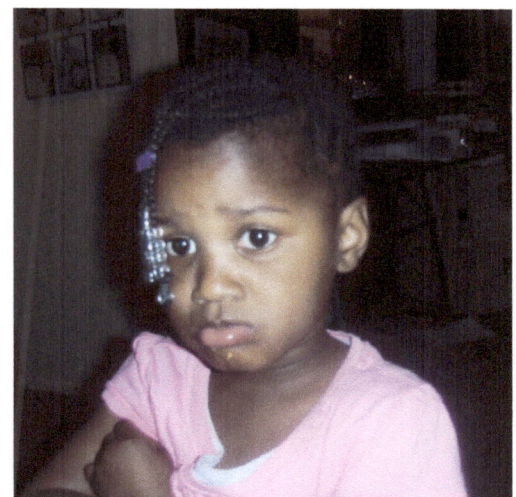

I'm not a rabbit.

Dd

Dandelions

English   Spanish

Four = 4   Cuatho = 4

Dandelions are wild plants grown in rural areas and farm locations. They supply vitamin A, C, and K. In the Eurasian countries they are cultivated for human consumption. The flower petals of dandelion are used to make dandelion wine and are one of the ingredients of root beer.

Some people consider dandelion a weed; some consider it a flower.

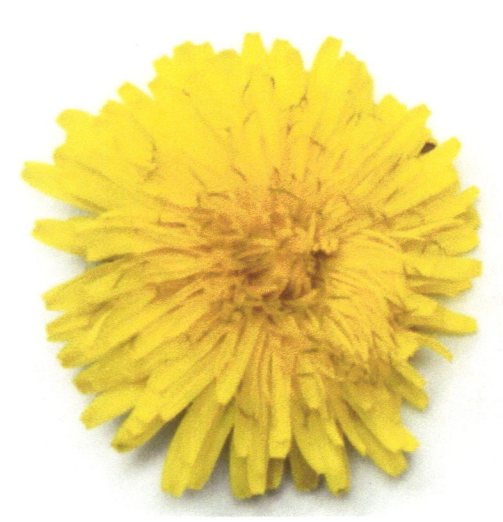

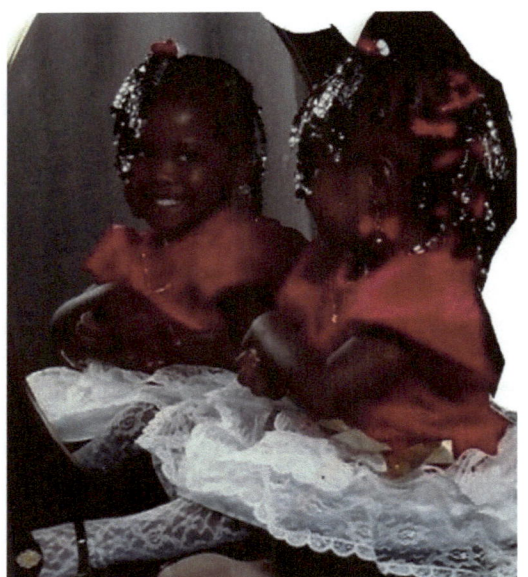

I'm full of myself.

Ee

Egg Plants

English	Spanish
Five = 5	Cinco = 5

Egg plants are used mostly for vegetarian and ethnic dishes. They are low in calories unless cooked in fat.

Which came first, the chicken or the egg plant?

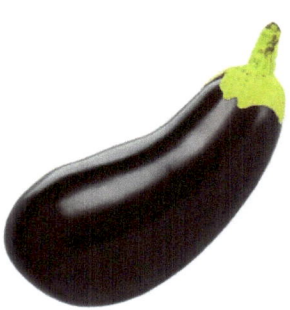

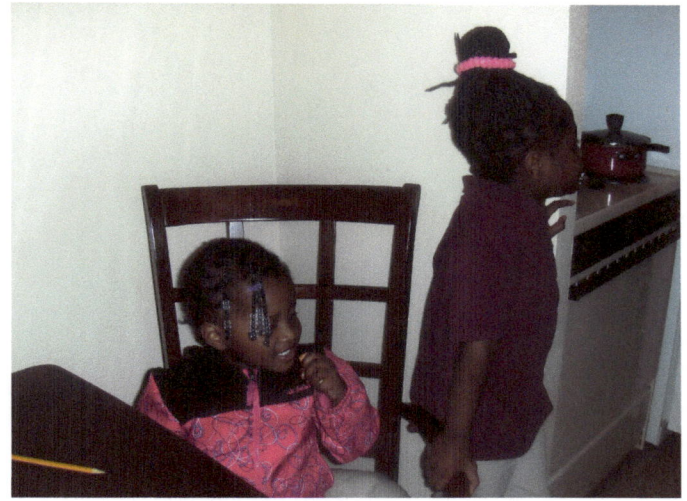

YUK!!!

Ff

Fennels

English   Spanish

Six = 6   Seis = 6

Fennels contain vitamins A and C, potassium, calcium, iron and fiber. The bulb, foliage and seeds are widely used in many of the culinary traditions of the world. For cooking, the bulb is a crisp vegetable that can be sautéed, stewed, braised, or eaten raw.

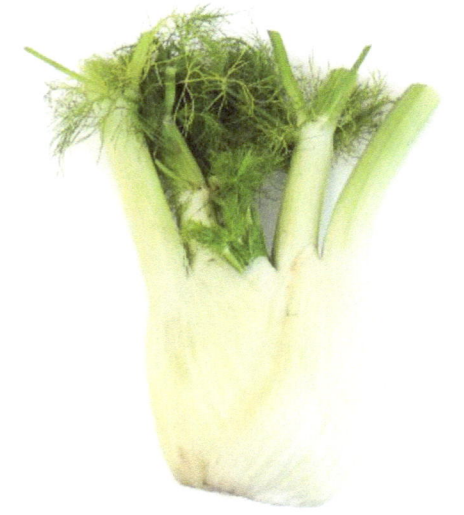

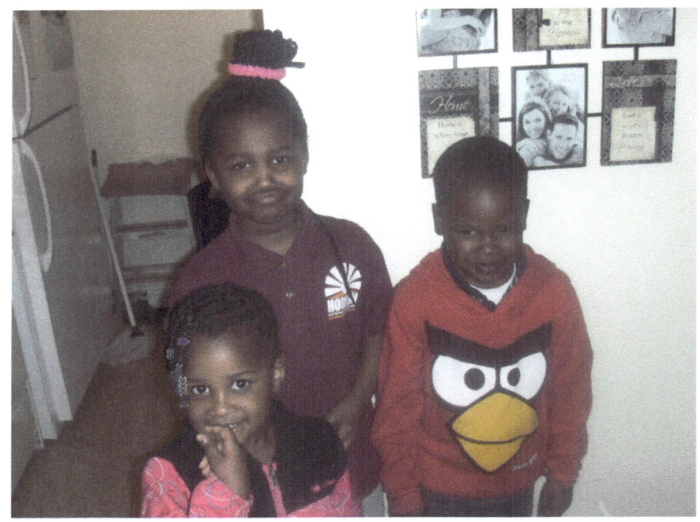

Enough! We protest.

Gg

Garlic

English	Spanish
Seven = 7	Siete = 7

Garlic is widely used around the world for its pungent flavor as a seasoning or condiment. Garlic bulbs are normally divided into numerous fleshy sections called cloves. These cloves are consumed (raw or cooked) or for medicinal purposes. Garlic can be applied to different kinds of bread to create a variety of classic dishes such as garlic bread, garlic toast, etc..

One of the drawbacks to eating garlic, of course, is that it causes "bad" breath (halitosis). But in 1924 it was found to prevent scurvy because of its high vitamin C content.

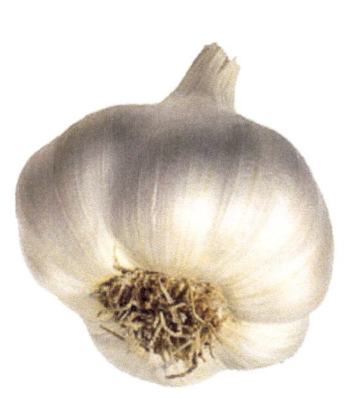

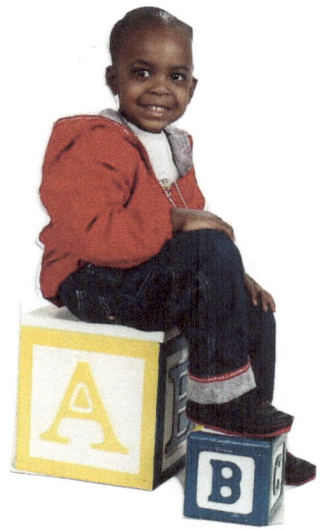

Bring it on, I'll eat it.

Hh

Habanero Peppers

English	Spanish
Eight = 8	Ocho =8

Habanero peppers are both hot and healthy. They are high in minerals and vitamins C and A. Capsaicin, the active "hot" chemical in habaneros, kills unwanted bacteria and intestinal parasites.

How hot is a habanero? A jalapeno pepper has an SHU (Scoville hot unit) of 5,000 and a habanero has an SHU of 200,000. That's hot.

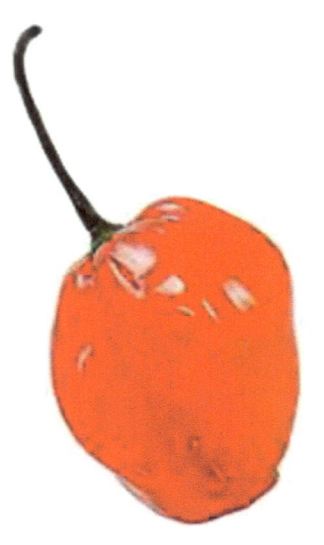

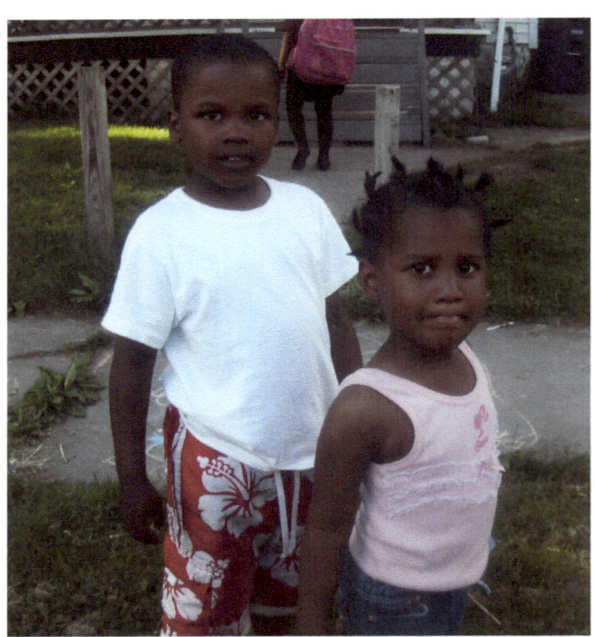

No way.

Ii

Indian Corn

English	Spanish
Nine = 9	Nueve = 9

Indian corn (flint corn) is one of three types of corn that was cultivated by Native Americans, both in New England and across the northern tier, including tribes such as the Pawnee on the Great Plains. Indian corn is the type of corn preferred for making hominy, and it is sometimes called "ornamental" corn because of its use in Thanksgiving decorations in the United States.

Because Indian corn has a very low water content it is more resistant to freezing than other vegetables. It was the only Vermont crop to survive New England's infamous "Year Without a Summer" of 1816.

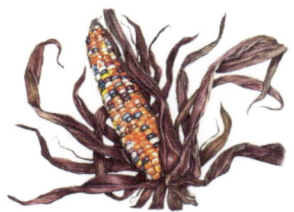

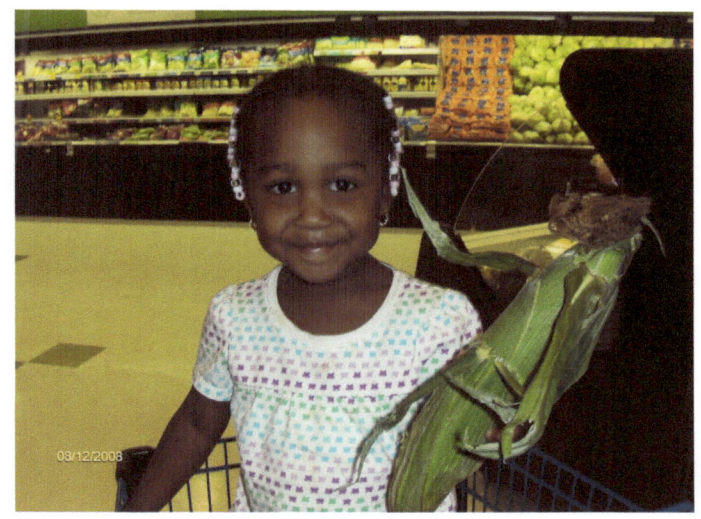

Corn?

Jj

Jack Beans

English   Spanish

Ten = 10   Diez = 10

Jack bean, canavalia ensiformis, is a legume which is used for animal fodder and human nutrition. In the United States, it is cultivated mainly in the southern states for animal fodder.

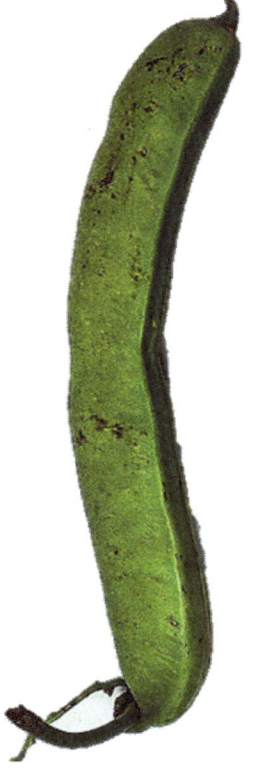

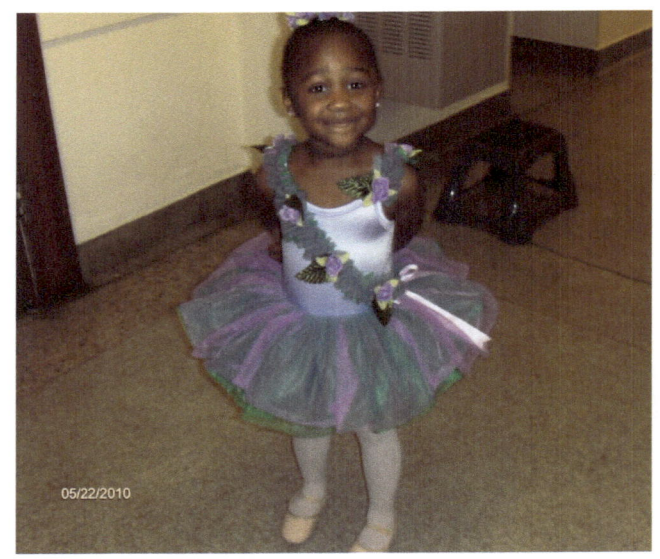

I want to be a dancer.

Kk

Kale

English   Spanish

Eleven = 11   Once = 11

Kale is a vegetable similar to cabbage, with green or purple leaves, in which the central leaves do not form a head. Kale is very high in beta carotene, vitamin K, C, and E, and is rich in calcium.

Kale freezes well and actually tastes sweeter and more flavorful after being exposed to frost.

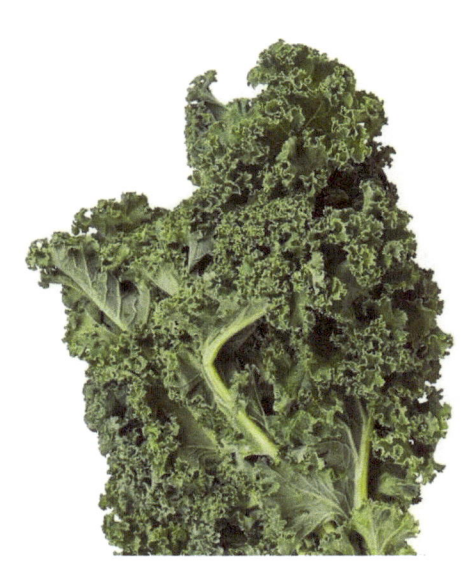

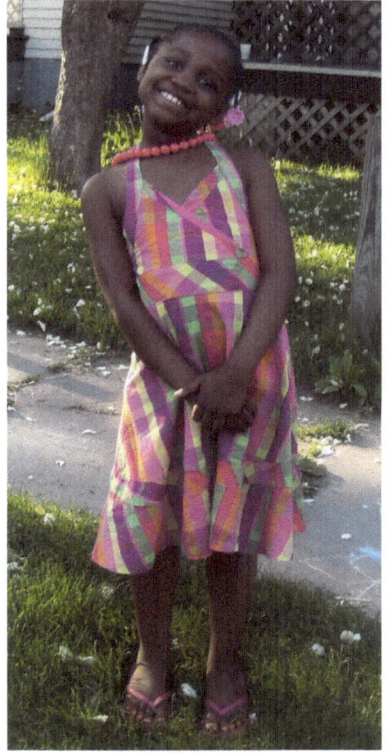

I'm cute.

Ll

Lettuce

English	Spanish
Twelve = 12	Doc = 12

Lettuce contains vitamin A, C, K, Calcium, Iron, and Potassium, with a higher concentration of vitamins found in darker green lettuce. Lettuce is most often used in salads, although it is also used in soups, sandwiches, and wraps.

Despite its beneficial properties, lettuce, when contaminated is often a source of bacterial, viral, and parasitic outbreaks in humans, including E. coli, and salmonella.

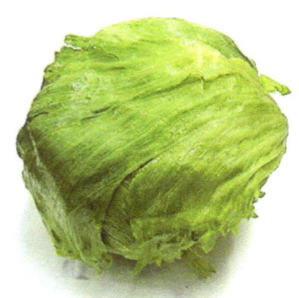

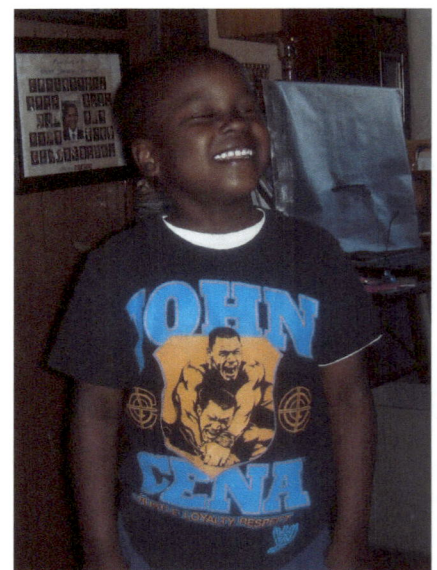

I'm bad!

Mm

Mushrooms

English   Spanish

Thirteen = 13   Trece = 13

Edible mushrooms are the fleshy and edible fruit bodies of several species of fungi.

Before assuming that any wild mushroom is edible it should be identified, because many species are very toxic to humans and can be very poisonous. As a rule all wild mushrooms should be cooked thoroughly before eating.

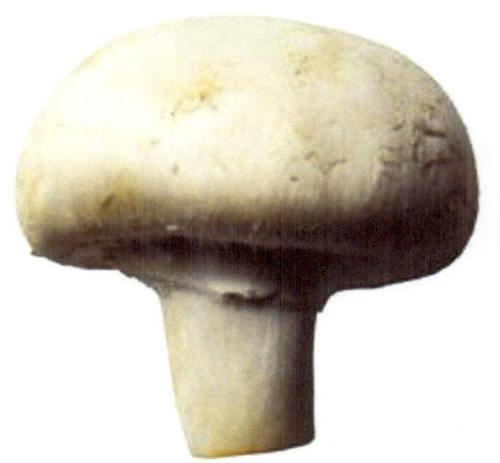

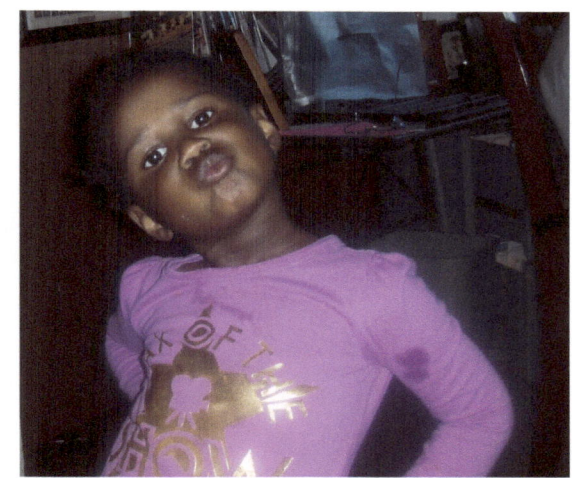

Mushrooms make me pucker.

Nn

Nectarine

English	Spanish
Fourteen = 14	Catorce = 14

A nectarine is rich in fiber, vitamin A, vitamin C, vitamin E, and potassium.

A nectarine has smooth skin and is sometimes called a "shaved peach" because of its lack of fuzz or short hairs. It is sometimes erroneously believed to be a cross between a peach and a plum. But though fuzzy peaches and nectarines are regarded commercially as different fruits, the nectarine is just a different species of peach.

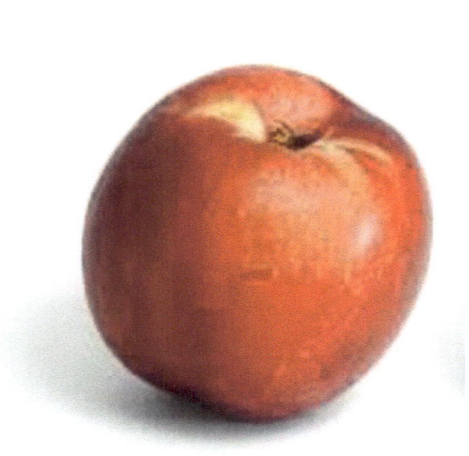

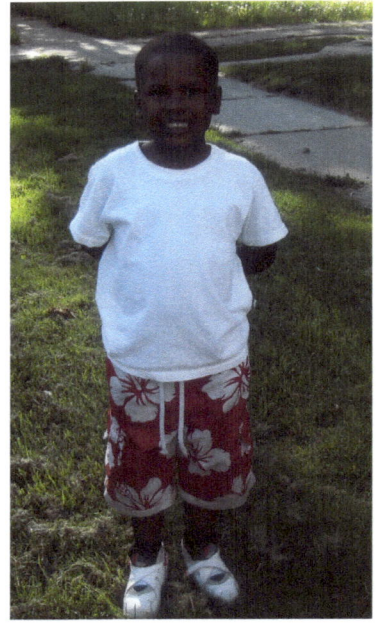

N-E-C-T-A-R-I-N-E

Oo

Onion

English   Spanish

Fifteen = 15   Decimoquinta = 15

Onions contain high amounts of vitamin C and are a good source of dietary fiber. They also contain chemical compounds such as phenolics and flavonoids that have potential anti-inflammatory, anti-cholesterol, anticancer and antioxidant properties.

In the Middle Ages onions were such an important food that people would pay their rent with onions, and even give them as gifts. According to diaries kept by early colonists in America, bulb onions were one of the first things planted by the Pilgrim Fathers when they cleared the land for cropping in 1648.

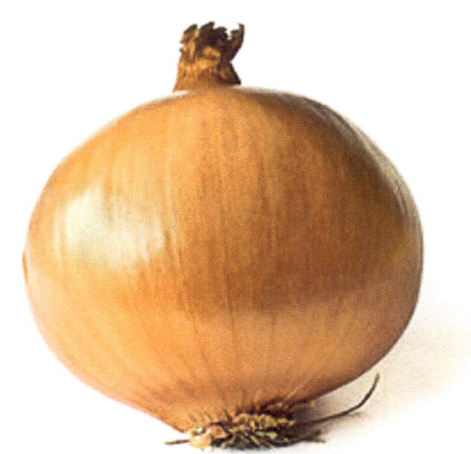
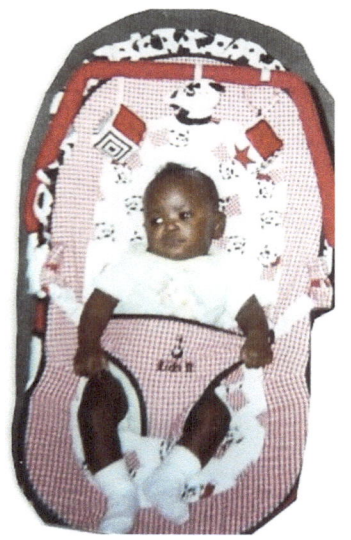

That was way before my time.

Pp

Potato

English	Spanish
Sixteen = 16	Dieciseis = 16

A medium sized potato with skin provides 27 mg of vitamin C (45 % of the daily value), and 620 mg of potassium (18 % of DV). The potato is best known for its carbohydrate content (about 26 grams in a medium potato).

Potatoes are the world's fourth-largest food crops, following rice, wheat, and maize (corn). Humans can survive healthily on a diet of potatoes supplemented only with milk or butter which contain the two vitamins not provided by potatoes: vitamin A and D.

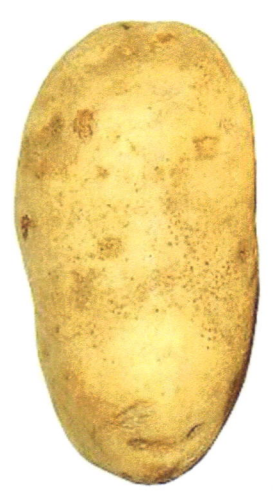 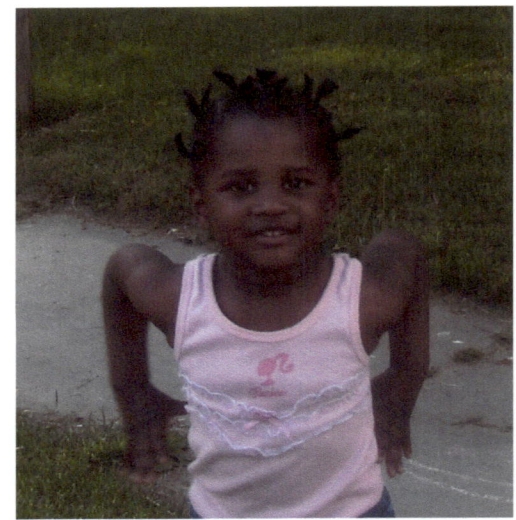

P-O-T-A-T-O

Qq

Quince

English	Spanish
Seventeen = 17	Diecisiete = 17

Quince is high in carbohydrates, vitamin C (18% DV), calcium, potassium, and dietary fiber. The U.S. gets most of its quince from Argtentina.

High in pectin, quince fruit is used to make jam and jelly. Originally, marmalade was made from quince fruit.

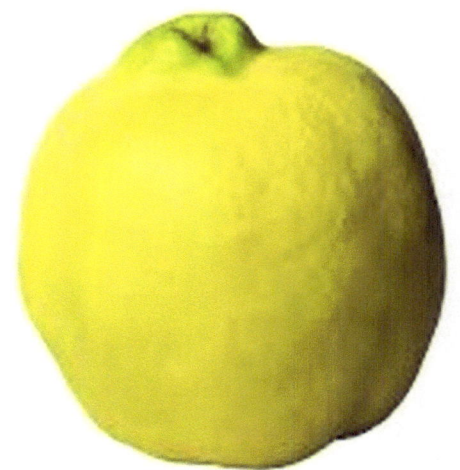

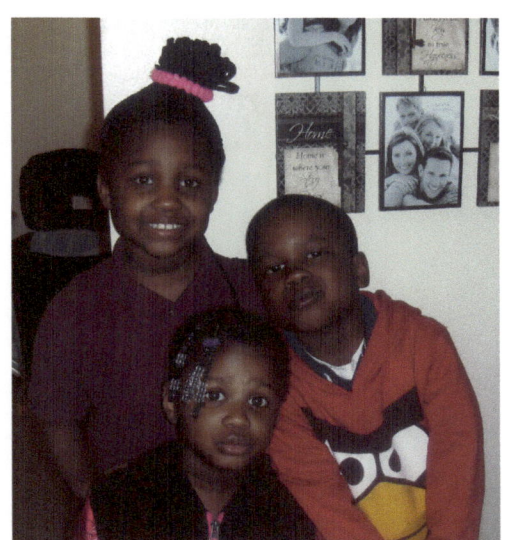

Is this where we get our jam and jelly?

Rr

Radish

English	Spanish
Eighteen = 18	Dieciocho = 18

Radishes are a good source of vitamin B6 and vitamin C, and are rich in ascorbic acid, folic acid, potassium and calcium. There are many varieties of radishes, but the most common radish seen in supermarkets in North America is the Cherry Belle, a bright red-skinned round variety.

The radish is a root plant; therefore insects can attack the leaves all day long with little effect on the edible root, which makes it a good companion plant for more vulnerable vegetables—sort of like a decoy.

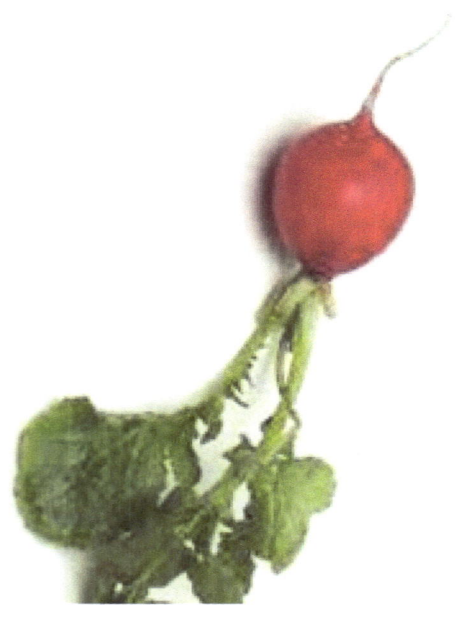

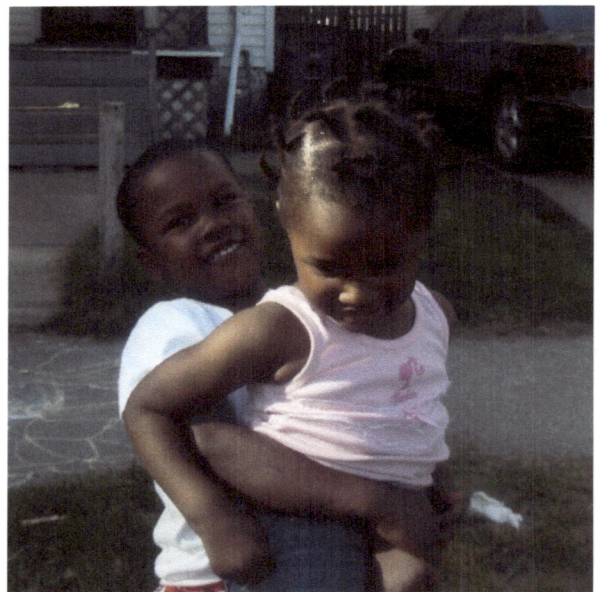

I've got muscles.

Ss

Squash

English   Spanish

Nineteen = 19   Diecinueve = 19

Squash is a source of many vitamins and minerals, with a high percentage of vitamin C (20%), vitamin B6 (17%) and riboflavin (12%).

Squash was one of the "Three Sisters" planted by Native Americans. These were the three main native crop plants: maize (corn), beans, and squash. They were usually planted together, with the corn stalk serving as support for the climbing beans, and shade for the squash.

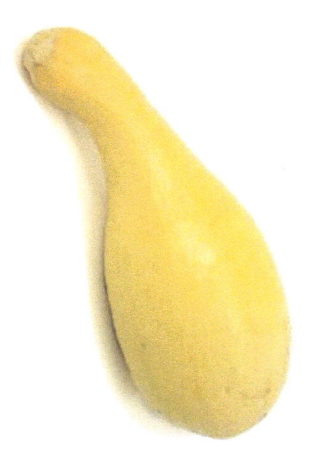

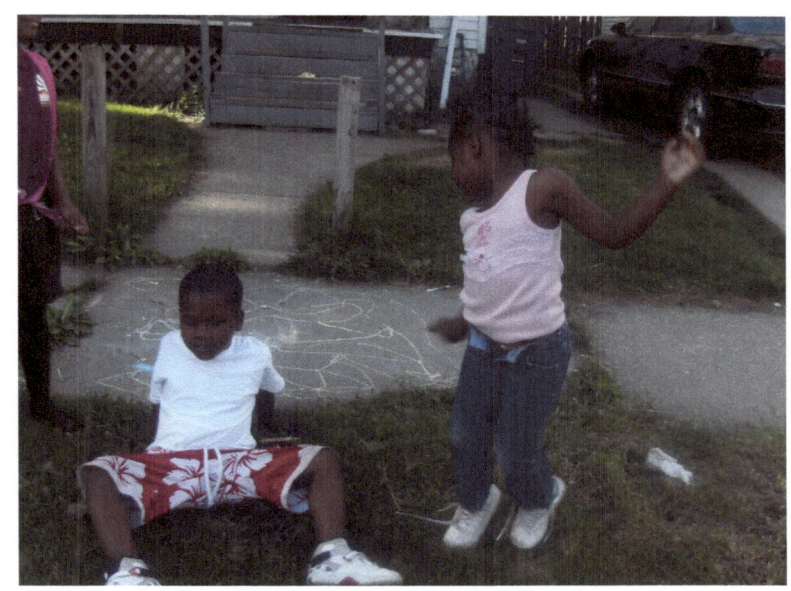

Oh yeah? Take that, big brother!

Tt

Tomato

English	Spanish
Twenty = 20	Veinte = 20

The tomato contains a powerful antioxidant, lycopene, and provides a high percentage of vitamin C, A, B6, and A, as well as many beneficial minerals such as potassium and manganese.

While the tomato is a fruit, it is considered a vegetable for culinary purposes. The Tariff Act of 1883 required a tax to be paid on imported vegetables but not fruit, so the U.S. Supreme Court ruled that the tomato should be classified under customs regulation as a vegetable instead of a fruit. Tricky stuff, huh? Botanically a tomato *is* a fruit because it is a seed-bearing structure growing from the flowering part of a plant.

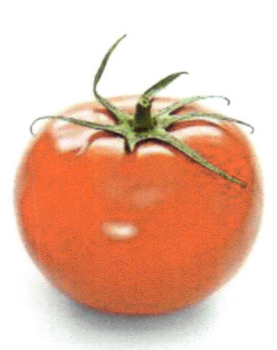

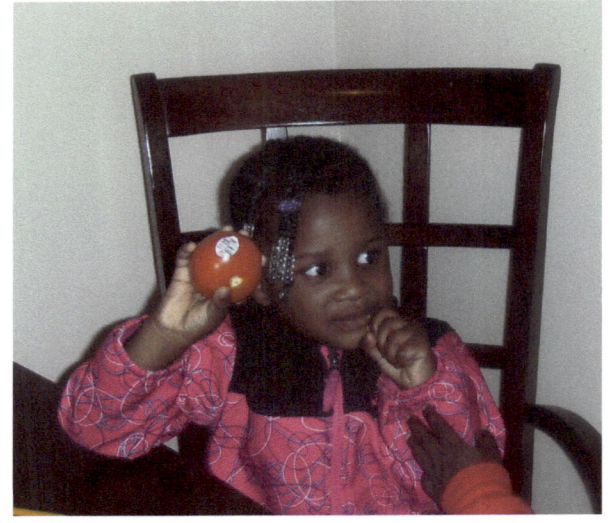

T-O-M-A-T-O

Uu

Ugli

English	Spanish
Twenty-one = 21	Veintiuno = 21

A single serving of Ugli fruit contains an amazing 70% of the recommended daily value of vitamin C to your diet.

UGLI is a trademark of Cold Hall Citrus Limited and under which it sells its Jamaican tangelo, a citrus fruit that is a cross between a grapefruit, an orange, and a tangerine. It was discovered growing wild in Jamaica by the people who, after an importer said, "…send me some more of that *ugly* fruit," changed its name to UGLI and developed it commercially.

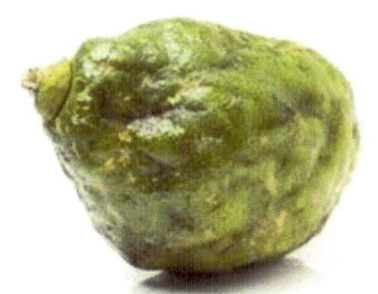
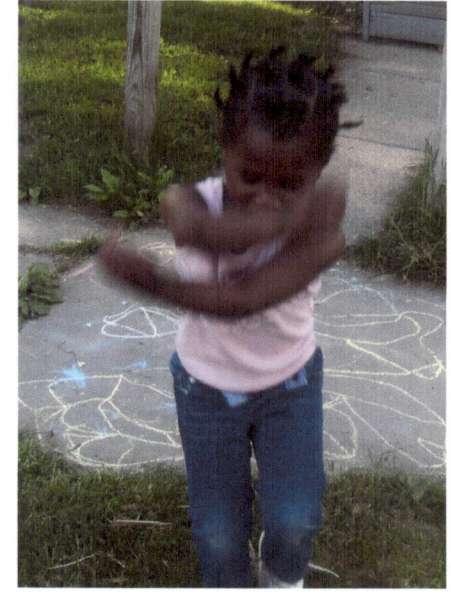

Phew!!! That's ugly.

Vv

Voavanga

English	Spanish
Twenty-two = 22	Veintidos = 22

Little is known in the United States about the nutritional value of the Voavanga (Spanish tamarind). It is said to be native to Mexico.

The Voavanga is a green round fruit with white dots. It turns brown when ripe.

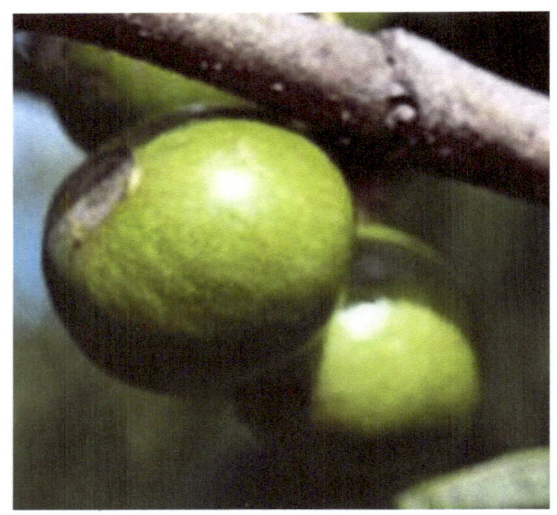

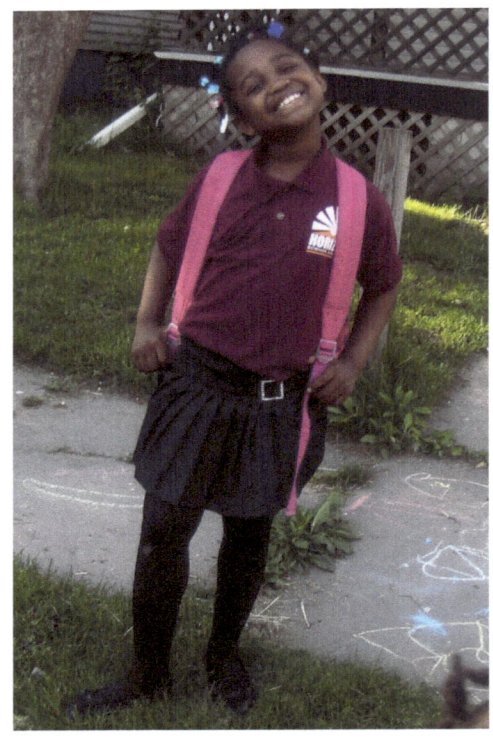

I-C-E C-R-E-A-M

Ww

Watermelon

English	Spanish
Twenty-three = 23	Veintitres = 23

A watermelon contains about 6% sugar and 91% water by weight, and like many other fruits it is a source of vitamin C (10% of daily requirements).

A lot of bees are required to pollinate a watermelon patch. The US Department of Agriculture recommends that for commercial planting one beehive per acre be provided for pollination of watermelons, and three beehives per acre for seedless watermelons because seedless varieties have sterile pollen.

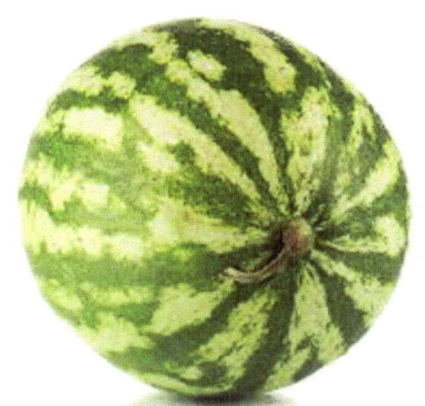

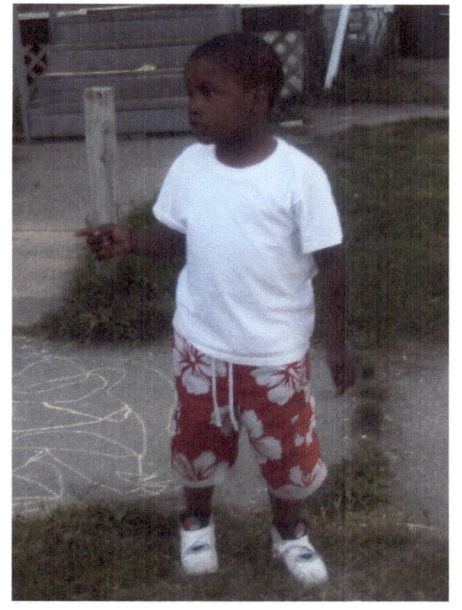

W-a-t-e-r-m-e-l-o-n

Xx

Xigua

English	Spanish
Twenty-four = 24	Veinticuatro = 24

Xigua is an African name for watermelon, the same watermelon pictured on the previous page, according to many sources. However, one source of information describes the xigua as an African melon like the watermelon except smaller and shorter in length. One fact they all agree on is that the watermelon, by whatever name, originated in Africa. Another fact we all can agree on is that the xigua starts with the letter X, thus fulfilling the alphabetical need of this book.

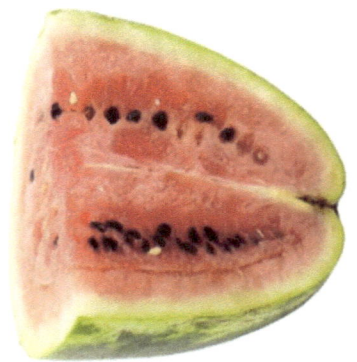

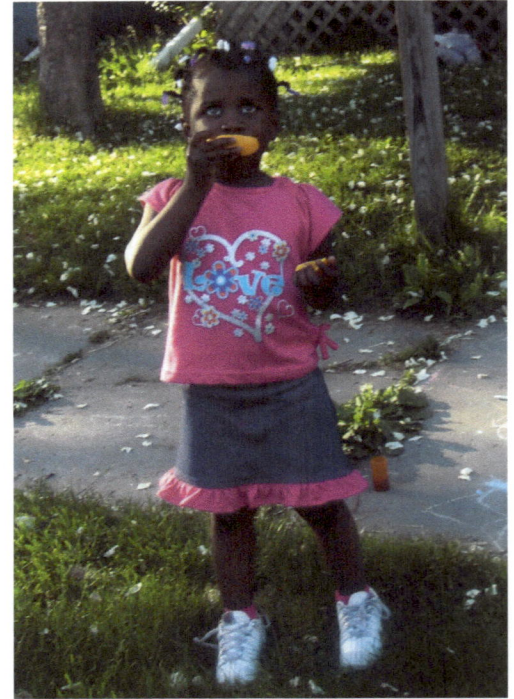

What about oranges, Granny?

Yy

Yams

English	Spanish
Twenty-five = 25	Veinticinco = 25

Yams (sweet potatoes) are rich in vitamins A, C, and B6, beta-carotene, and potassium. In 1992 the nutritional value of sweet potatoes was compared to other vegetables. Considering fiber content, complex carbohydrates, protein, vitamins A and C, iron and calcium, the sweet potato was the highest in nutritional value with a score of 184, more than a hundred points higher than the next on the list, the common potato.

Yams are native to Africa, where 95% of them are grown. They are not sweet potatoes. However, the "soft" varieties of sweet potatoes are often called yams in the United States. So if you are eating a yam in the U.S. you are probably eating a sweet potato.

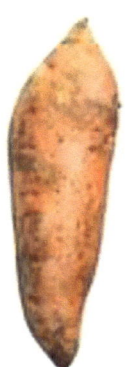

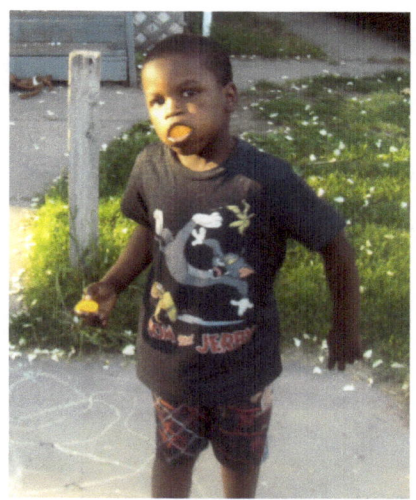

Yes, I vote for oranges, too.

Zz

Zucchini

English	Spanish
Twenty-six = 26	Veintiseis = 26

The zucchini squash is low in calories. It contains significant amounts of folate, potassium, and vitamin A.

The zucchini squash is a fruit; however it is treated as a vegetable for culinary purposes. While easy to grow, zucchini, like all squash, requires plentiful bees for pollination.

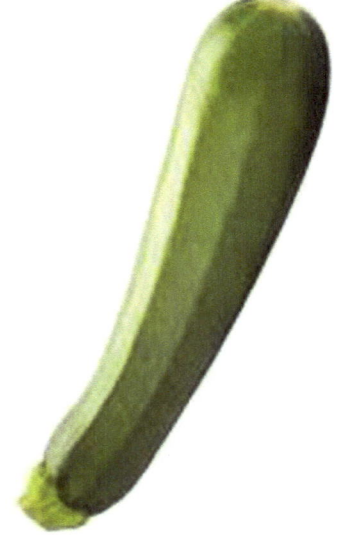

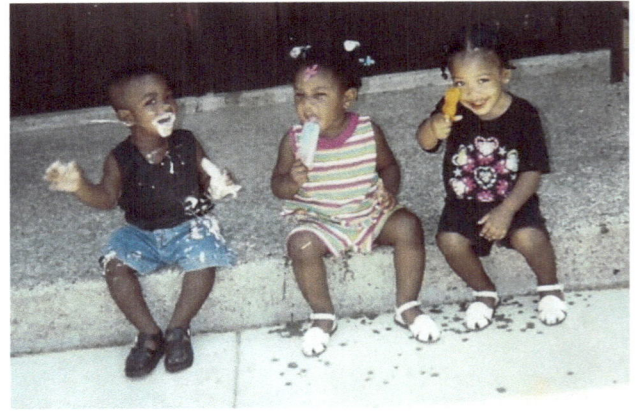

Hey!!! It is a great day!!!
Reward Day!!!

Our acknowledgement of the wealth of information we gathered from Wikipedia online encyclopedia and Vox New College Spanish and English Dictionary Second Edition.

And, of course, many thanks to Google.

ISBN-13: 978-1490905266
ISBN-10: 149090526X

www.ingramcontent.com/pod-product-compliance
Lightning Source LLC
Chambersburg PA
CBHW060810290526
45792CB00005BA/1600